Anti-Inflammatory Meat Cookbook

50+ Meat Recipes to Heal your Body for a healthy life

Natalie Worley

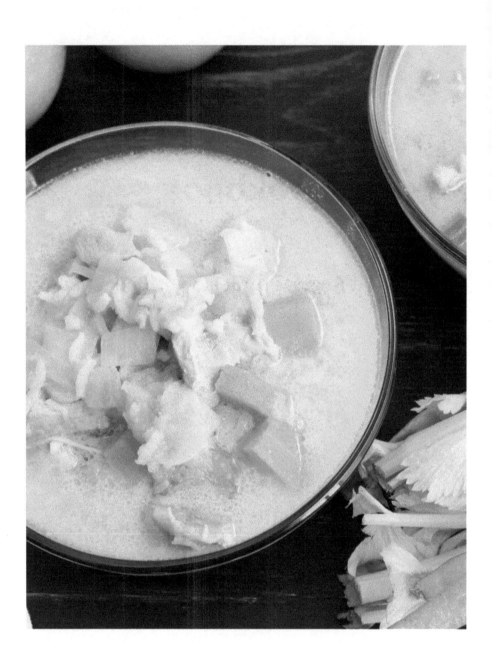

any techniques outlined in this book.

by reading this document, the reader agrees that under no circumstances is the author responsible for any losses, direct or indirect, which are incurred as a result of the use of information contained within this document, including, but not limited to, — errors, omissions, or inaccuracies.

Table of Contents

Chicken Mulligatawny

Prep Time: 35 minutes | **Serve:** 4

- 2 tablespoons ghee
- 1 pound chicken thighs, boneless and skinless
- 1 tablespoon Indian spice mix
- 1 celery stalk, chopped
- 1 cup milk

1.Melt the butter in a soup pot over medium-high flame. Brown the chicken thighs until nicely browned on all sides about 6 minutes.

2.Add in Indian spice mix and celery; stir to combine and reduce the heat to simmer; continue to simmer for 30 minutes more.

3.Pour in the milk and stir to combine well. Bon appétit!

Nutrition: 343 Calories; 26.7g Fat; 3.8g Carbs; 20.9g

Protein; 0.2g Fiber

Naga Chicken Salad Ole

Prep Time: 20 minutes + chilling time | **Serve:** 6

- 1/2 cup dry white wine

- 1 ½ pounds chicken breasts

- 1 Spanish naga chili pepper, chopped

- 1/4 cup mayonnaise

- 2 cups arugula

1.Place the chicken breasts and wine in a deep saucepan.

Then, cover the chicken with water, and bring to a boil.

2.When your mixture reaches boiling, reduce the

temperature to a simmer.

3.Let it simmer, partially covered, for about 13 minutes

or until cooked through.

4.Shred the chicken, discarding the bones and poaching liquid. Place in a salad bowl and add naga chili pepper, arugula, and mayonnaise to the bowl.

5.Add Spanish peppers, if desired and stir to combine well.

Nutrition: 278 Calories; 16.1g Fat; 4.9g Carbs; 27.2g Protein; 0.9g Fiber

Oven-Roasted Chimichurri Chicken

Prep Time: 40 minutes + marinating time | **Serve:** 5

- 1 ½ pounds chicken tenders
- ½ cup fresh parsley, chopped
- 2 garlic cloves, minced
- ¼ cup olive oil
- 4 tablespoons white wine vinegar

1.Blend the parsley, olive oil, vinegar, and garlic in your food processor until the smooth and uniform sauce forms. Pierce the chicken with a small knife.

2.Add chicken and 1/2 of the chimichurri sauce to a glass dosh and let them marinate for 2 hours in your refrigerator.

3.Spritz a baking pan with nonstick cooking spray. Place the chicken in the baking pan. Season with salt and black pepper.

4.Bake in the preheated oven at 360 degrees F for 35 minutes or until an internal temperature reaches about 165 degrees F.

5.Serve with the reserved chimichurri sauce. Bon appétit!

Nutrition: 305 Calories; 14.7g Fat; 0.8g Carbs; 27.9g Protein; 0.2g Fiber

Classic Garlicky Chicken Drumettes

Prep Time: 40 minutes + marinating time | **Serve:** 5

¼ cup coconut aminos

1 tablespoon olive oil

1 tablespoon apple cider vinegar

2 cloves garlic, minced

5 chicken drumettes

1.Thoroughly combine, coconut aminos, olive oil, apple cider vinegar, and garlic in a glass dish. Allow it to marinate for 2 hours in your refrigerator

2.Place the chicken in a foil-lined baking dish. Season with salt and black pepper to taste.

3.Bake in the preheated oven at 410 degrees F for 35 minutes, basting the chicken with the reserved marinade.

Nutrition: 266 Calories; 19.3g Fat; 0.8g Carbs; 20.3g Protein; 0.2g Fiber

Barbeque Chicken Wings

Prep Time: 15 min | **Cook Time:** 14 min | **Serve:** 6

- 2 lb. chicken wings

- ½ teaspoon basil; dried

- ¾ cup BBQ sauce

- 1 teaspoon red pepper; crushed.

- 2 teaspoons paprika

- Salt and black pepper to the taste

1.Start by tossing the chicken wings with remaining ingredients in a bowl.

2.Prepare and preheat a grill to cook the wings.

3.Grill the wings for 7 minutes per side on medium low heat.

Nutrition: Calories 251, Total Fat 15.3 g, Saturated Fat 6.5 g, Cholesterol 122 mg, Sodium 366 mg, Total Carbs 3 g, Fiber 1.8 g, Sugar 0.9 g, Protein 25 g

Saucy Duck

Prep Time: 15 min | **Cook Time:** 15 min | **Serve:** 2

- 1 duck, cut into small chunks

- 2 tablespoon ginger garlic paste

- 2 green onions; roughly chopped

- 4 tablespoon soy sauce

- 4 tablespoon sherry wine

- Salt and black pepper to the taste

1.Start by tossing the duck with all other ingredients in a bowl.

2.Marinate the meat for 4 hours in the refrigerator.

3.Spread the duck chunks in a baking tray.

4.Bake the meat for 15 minutes with occasional tossing.

Nutrition: Calories 225, Total Fat 14.3 g, Saturated Fat 0.6 g, Cholesterol 137 mg, Sodium 538 mg, Total Carbs 2.8 g, Fiber 7 g, Sugar 0.3 g, Protein 28.2 g

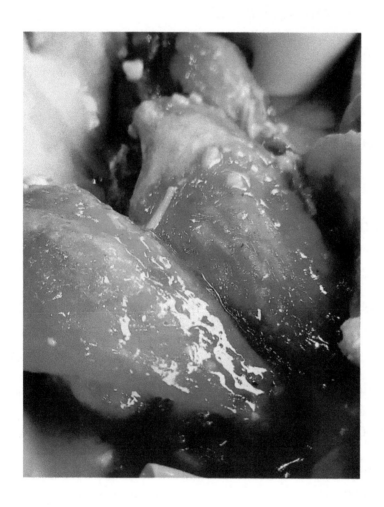

Chicken Roux Gumbo

Prep Time: 15 min | **Cook Time:** 20 min | **Serve:** 2

- 1 lb. chicken thighs; cut into halves
- ¼ cup 1 tablespoon vegetable oil 1/2 cup almond flour
- 1 cup vegetable stock
- 1 teaspoon Cajun spice
- Salt and black pepper to the taste

1.Start by toss the chicken with salt, black pepper and 1 tablespoon oil in a bowl.

2.Cover the thighs and refrigerate for 1 hour for marination.

3.Sear the marinated chicken in a sauté pan.

4.Cook for 5 minutes per side until golden brown.

5.Whisk almond flour with Cajun spice and remaining oil in a separate bowl.

6.Add almond mixture to a cooking pot and stir cook for 2 minutes.

7.Stir in stock and cook well until it thickens.

8.Toss in the sear chicken and cook for 4 minutes.

Nutrition: Calories 433, Total Fat 15.2 g, Saturated Fat 8.6 g, Cholesterol 179 mg, Sodium 318 mg, Total Carbs 2.7 g, Fiber 1.1 g, Sugar 1.1 g, Protein 68.4 g

Chunky Salsa Chicken

Prep Time: 15 min | **Cook Time:** 25 min | **Serve:** 2

- 1 lb. chicken breast, skinless and boneless

- 1 cup chunky salsa

- ¾ teaspoon cumin

- A pinch of oregano

- Salt and black pepper to the taste

1. Pat dry the chicken and rub it with salt and pepper.

2. Place this chicken in the insert of the Instant Pot.

3. Add cumin, oregano and chunky salsa.

4. Mix well then seal the lid of the Instant Pot.

5. Cook on poultry mode for 25 minutes.

6. Once done, release the pressure quickly then shred meat with a fork.

7.Serve the meat with its salsa.

Nutrition: Calories 272, Total Fat 27 g, Saturated Fat 16 g, Cholesterol 83 mg, Sodium 175 mg, Total Carbs 7.8 g, Fiber 0.4 g, Sugar 5.2 g, Protein 5.3 g

Dijon Chicken

Prep Time: 15 min | **Cook Time:** 20 min | **Serve:** 6

- 2 lb. chicken thighs; skinless and boneless 1/4 cup lemon juice
- 2 tablespoon extra-virgin olive oil
- 3 tablespoon Dijon mustard
- 2 tablespoon Italian seasoning
- Salt and black pepper to the taste

1.Start by tossing chicken with all other ingredients in a bowl.

2.Prepare and preheat the grill on medium heat.

3.Grill the chicken pieces for 5 minutes per side until al dente.

Nutrition: Calories 242, Total Fat 15.9 g, Saturated Fat 10.6 g, Cholesterol 36 mg, Sodium 421 mg, Total Carbs 4.6 g, Fiber 2 g, Sugar 1.6 g, Protein 20.8 g

Chicken Thighs with Vegetables

Prep Time: 15 min | **Cook Time:** 30 min | **Serve:** 6s

- 6 chicken thighs

- 15 oz. canned tomatoes; chopped.

- 1 yellow onion; chopped.

- 2 cups chicken stock

- 1/4 lb. baby carrots; cut into halves

- Salt and black pepper to the taste

1.Start by adding chicken and all other ingredients to a cooking pot.

2.Cove the pot's lid and cook for 30 minutes on medium low heat.

3.Mix well and serve fresh.

Nutrition: Calories 362, Total Fat 15.9 g, Saturated Fat 9.9 g, Cholesterol 49 mg, Sodium 684 mg, Total Carbs 4.1 g, Fiber 1.4 g, Sugar 1.1 g, Protein 23.3 g

Chicken Dipped in Tomatillo Sauce

Prep Time: 15 min | **Cook Time:** 15 min | **Serve:** 2

- 1 lb. chicken thighs; skinless and boneless
- 2 tablespoon extra-virgin olive oil
- 1 yellow onion; thinly sliced
- 5 oz. tomatoes; chopped.
- Salt and black pepper to the taste
- 15 oz. canned tomatillos; chopped.

1.Start by heating olive oil in a cooking pot.

2.Toss in chicken, tomatillos, onion, salt, pepper, and tomatoes.

3.Cook for 15 minutes on medium low heat and cover the

pot's lid.

4.Stir well and serve fresh.

Nutrition: Calories 260, Total Fat 13 g, Saturated Fat 5

g, Cholesterol 0.3 mg, Sodium 465 mg, Total Carbs 6 g,

Fiber 5.4 g, Sugar 1.3 g, Protein 26 g

Crispy Italian Chicken

Prep Time: 15 min | **Cook Time:** 10 min | **Serve:** 6

- 6 chicken thighs

- 1 cup almond flour

- 2 eggs; whisked

- 1 ½ cups panko breadcrumbs

- Salt and black pepper to the taste

1.Start by tossing the flour with salt and black pepper in a flat plate.

2.Whisk the eggs in a separate bowl and spread breadcrumbs in a plate.

3.Coat the chicken thighs with the flour then dip in the eggs and then coat with crumbs.

4.Prepare and preheat the grill on medium heat.

5.Grill the chicken for 5 minutes per side on medium heat.

Nutrition: Calories 355, Total Fat 16.8 g, Saturated Fat 4 g, Cholesterol 150 mg, Sodium 719 mg, Total Carbs 1.4 g, Fiber 0.5 g, Sugar 0.1 g, Protein 47 g

Cacciatore Olive Chicken

Prep Time: 15 min | **Cook Time:** 20 min | **Serve:** 8

- 28 oz. canned tomatoes and juice; crushed.

- 8 chicken drumsticks; bone-in

- ½ cup olives; pitted and sliced

- 1 cup chicken stock

- 1 yellow onion; chopped.

- Salt and black pepper, to the taste

1.Start by adding chicken and all other ingredients to a cooking pot.

2.Cover the pot's lid and cook for 20 minutes with occasional stirring.

Nutrition: Calories 489, Total Fat 18.7 g, Saturated Fat 3.8 g, Cholesterol 151 mg, Sodium 636 mg, Total Carbs 6.1 g, Fiber 0.5 g, Sugar 4.3 g, Protein 50 g

Duck and Vegetable Stew

Prep Time: 15 min | **Cook Time:** 40 min | **Serve:** 6

- 1 duck; chopped into medium pieces

- 2 carrots; chopped

- 2 cups of water

- 1 cucumber; chopped

- 1-inch ginger pieces; chopped

- Salt and black pepper to the taste

1.Place the duck pieces in the Instant Pot Add carrots, wine, ginger, water, salt, and pepper.

2.Mix well and seal the lid. Cook for 40 minutes on Poultry mode.

3.Once done, release the pressure quickly, then remove the lid.

Nutrition: Calories 325, Total Fat 14.4 g, Saturated Fat 3.5 g, Cholesterol 135 mg, Sodium 552 mg, Total Carbs 2.3 g, Fiber 0.4 g, Sugar 0.5 g, Protein 44 g

Chicken Eggplant Curry

Prep Time: 15 min | **Cook Time:** 15 min | **Serve:** 4

- 8 chicken pieces

- 1 eggplant; cubed

- 3 garlic cloves; crushed.

- 14 oz. canned coconut milk

- 2 tablespoon green curry paste

- Salt and black pepper to the taste

1.Start by adding chicken and all other ingredients to a cooking pot.

2.Cover the pot's lid and cook for 15 minutes with occasional stirring.

Nutrition: Calories 452, Total Fat 3.5 g, Saturated Fat 0.5 g, Cholesterol 181 mg, Sodium 461 mg, Total Carbs 7.5 g, Fiber 1.7 g, Sugar 1.3 g, Protein 91.8 g

Mushroom Cream Goose Curry

Prep Time: 15 min |**Cook Time:** 25 min | **Serve:** 4

- 12 oz. canned mushroom cream

- 3 goose breasts; fat trimmed off and cut into pieces

- 1 yellow onion; chopped.

- 3 ½ cups water

- 2 teaspoon garlic; minced.

- Salt and black pepper to the taste

1.Start by adding chicken and all other ingredients to a cooking pot.

2.Cover the pot's lid and cook for 25 minutes with occasional stirring.

Nutrition: Calories 386, Total Fat 10 g, Saturated Fat 1.7 g, Cholesterol 93 mg, Sodium 179 mg, Total Carbs 11.7 g, Fiber 0.4 g, Sugar 0.7 g, Protein 25.7 g

Chicken Curry

Prep Time: 15 min | **Cook Time:** 25 min | **Serve:** 8

- 3 lb. chicken drumsticks and thighs
- 1 yellow onion; finely chopped
- 1 cup chicken stock
- 15 oz. canned tomatoes; crushed.
- 1 lb. spinach; chopped.
- Salt and black pepper to the taste

1.Start by adding chicken and all other ingredients to a cooking pot.

2.Cover the pot's lid and cook for 25 minutes with occasional stirring.

Nutrition: Calories 283, Total Fat 23 g, Saturated Fat 7.9 g, Cholesterol 69 mg, Sodium 106 mg, Total Carbs 0.2 g, Fiber 0.1 g, Sugar 0 g, Protein 18 g

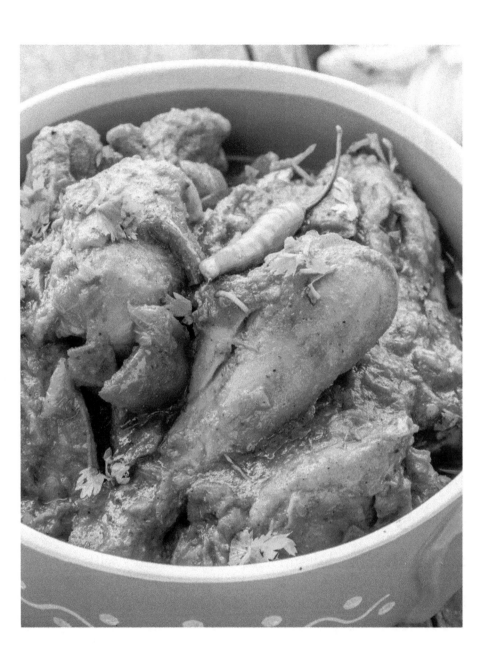

Saucy Teriyaki Chicken

Prep Time: 15 min | **Cook Time:** 25 min | **Serve:** 4

- 2 lb. chicken breasts; skinless and boneless, diced

- 1 cup teriyaki sauce

- ½ cup chicken stock

- A handful green onions; chopped.

- Salt and black pepper to the taste

1.Start by adding chicken and all other ingredients to a cooking pot.

2.Cover the pot's lid and cook for 25 minutes with occasional stirring.

Nutrition: Calories 402, Total Fat 20.8 g, Saturated Fat 5 g, Cholesterol 130 mg, Sodium 112 mg, Total Carbs 2.9 g, Fiber 0.9 g, Sugar 0.8 g, Protein 50.5 g

Chicken Shrimp Curry

Prep Time: 15 min | **Cook Time:** 20 min | **Serve:** 2

- 8 oz. shrimp; peeled and deveined
- 8 oz. chicken breasts; skinless; boneless and chopped.
- 2 tablespoon extra-virgin olive oil
- 2 teaspoon Creole seasoning
- 1 cup chicken stock
- 2 cups canned tomatoes; chopped.

1.Start by adding chicken and all other ingredients except shrimp to a cooking pot.

2.Cover the pot's lid and cook for 15 minutes with occasional stirring.

3.Toss in shrimp and cook for another 5 minutes.

Nutrition: Calories 377, Total Fat 11.4 g, Saturated Fat 1.8 g, Cholesterol 168 mg, Sodium 215 mg, Total Carbs 10.4 g, Fiber 0.2 g, Sugar 0.1 g, Protein 64 g

Whole Chicken with Prunes and Capers

Prep Time: 55 minutes | **Serve:** 6

- 1 whole chicken, 3 lb
- ½ cup pitted prunes
- 3 minced cloves of garlic
- 2 tbsp capers
- 2 bay leaves
- 2 tbsp red wine vinegar
- 2 tbsp olive oil
- 1 tbsp dried oregano
- ¼ cup packed brown sugar
- 1 tbsp chopped and fresh parsley
- Salt and black pepper

1.In a big and deep bowl, mix the prunes, the olives, capers, garlic, olive oil, bay leaves, oregano, vinegar, salt and pepper. Spread the mixture on the bottom of a baking tray, and place the chicken.

2.Preheat the Air Fryer to 360 F. Sprinkle a little bit of brown sugar on top of the chicken; cook for 55 minutes.

White Wine Chicken with Herbs

Prep Time: 45 minutes | **Serve:** 6

- 1 whole chicken, around 3 lb, cut in pieces
- 3 chopped cloves of garlic
- ½ cup olive oil
- ½ cup white wine
- 1 tbsp fresh rosemary
- 1 tbsp chopped fresh oregano
- 1 tbsp fresh thyme
- Juice from 1 lemon
- Salt and black pepper, to taste

1.In a large bowl, combine cloves of garlic, rosemary,

thyme, olive oil, lemon juice, oregano, salt and pepper.

Mix all ingredients very well and spread the mixture into

a baking dish. Add the chicken and stir.

2.Preheat the Air Fryer to 380 F, and transfer in the

chicken mixture. Sprinkle with wine and cook for 45

minutes.

Tasty Chicken Quarters with Broccoli & Rice

Prep Time: 60 minutes | **Serve:** 3

- 3 chicken leg quarters

- 1 package instant long grain rice

- 1 cup chopped broccoli

- 2 cups water

- 1 can condensed cream chicken soup

- 1 tbsp minced garlic

1.Preheat the Air Fryer to 390 F, and place the chicken quarters in the Air Fryer. Season with salt, pepper and one tbsp of oil; cook for 30 minutes. Meanwhile, in a large deep bowl, mix the rice, water, minced garlic, soup and broccoli. Combine the mixture very well.

2.Remove the chicken from the Air fryer and place it on a platter to drain. Spread the rice mixture on the bottom of the dish and place the chicken on top of the rice. Cook again for 30 minutes.

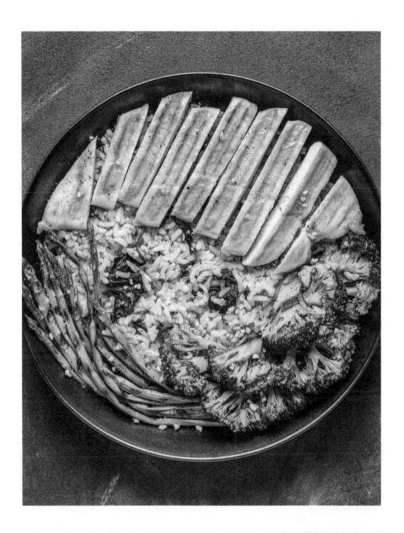

Asian-style Chicken with Vegetables

Prep Time: 35 minutes | **Serve:** 4

- 1 lb chicken, cut in stripes

- 2 tomatoes, cubed

- 3 green peppers, cut in stripes

- 1 tbsp cumin powder

- 1 large onion

- 2 tbsp oil

- 1 tbsp mustard

- A pinch of ginger

- A pinch of fresh and chopped coriander

- Salt and black pepper

1.Heat the oil in a deep pan. Add the mustard, the onion, the ginger, the cumin and the green chili peppers. Sauté the mixture for 2-3 minutes. Then, add the tomatoes, the coriander and salt and keep stirring.

2.Preheat the Air Fryer to 380 F. Coat the chicken with oil, salt and pepper and cook it for 25 minutes. Remove from the Air Fryer and pour the sauce over and around.

Southwest-Style Buttermilk Chicken Thighs

Prep Time: 4 hrs 40 minutes | **Serve:** 6

- 1 ½ lb chicken thighs
- 1 tbsp cayenne pepper
- 3 tbsp salt divided
- 2 cups flour
- 2 tbsp black pepper
- 1 tbsp paprika
- 1 tbsp baking powder
- 2 cups buttermilk

1.Rinse and pat dry the chicken thighs. Place the chicken thighs in a bowl. Add cayenne pepper, 2 tbsp of salt, black pepper and buttermilk, and stir to coat well.

Refrigerate for 4 hours. Preheat the air fryer to 350 F.

2.In another bowl, mix the flour, paprika, 1 tbsp of salt,

and baking powder. Dredge half of the chicken thighs,

one at a time, in the flour, and then place on a lined dish.

Cook for 10 minutes, flip over and cook for 8 more

minutes. Repeat with the other batch.

Coconut Crunch Chicken Strips

Prep Time: 22 minutes | **Serve:** 4

- 3 ½ cups coconut flakes

- 4 chicken breasts cut into strips

- ½ cup cornstarch ¼ tsp pepper

- ¼ tsp salt

- 3 eggs, beaten

1.Preheat the Air fryer to 350 F. Mix salt, pepper, and cornstarch in a small bowl. Line a baking sheet with parchment paper. Dip the chicken first in the cornstarch, then into the eggs, and finally, coat with coconut flakes. Arrange on the sheet and cook for 8 minutes. Flip the chicken over, and cook for 8 more minutes, until crispy.

American-Style Buttermilk

Fried Chicken

Prep Time: 30 minutes | **Serve:** 4

- 6 chicken drumsticks, skin on and bone in

- 2 cups buttermilk

- 2 tbsp salt

- 2 tbsp black pepper

- 1 tbsp cayenne pepper

- 2 cups all-purpose flour

- 1 tbsp baking powder

- 1 tbsp garlic powder

- 1 tbsp paprika

- 1 tbsp salt

1.Rinse chicken thoroughly underwater and pat them dry; remove any fat residue. In a large bowl, mix paprika, black pepper and chicken. Toss well to coat the chicken evenly. Pour buttermilk over chicken and toss to coat.

2.Let the chicken chill overnight. Preheat your Air Fryer to 400 F. In another bowl, mix flour, paprika, pepper and salt. Roll the chicken in the seasoned flour. Place the chicken in the cooking basket in a single layer and cook for 10 minutes. Repeat the same steps for the other pieces.

Chicken With Parmesan and Sage

Prep Time: 12 minutes | **Serve:** 4

- 4 chicken breasts, skinless and boneless
- 3 oz breadcrumbs
- 2 tbsp grated Parmesan cheese
- 2 oz flour
- 2 eggs, beaten
- 1 tbsp fresh, chopped sage

1.Preheat the air fryer to 370 F. Place some plastic wrap underneath and on top of the chicken breasts. Using a rolling pin, beat the meat until it becomes really thin. In a bowl, combine the Parmesan cheese, sage and breadcrumbs.

2.Dip the chicken in the egg first, and then in the sage mixture. Spray with cooking oil and arrange the meat in the air fryer. Cook for 7 minutes.

Party Chicken Tenders

Prep Time: 25 minutes | **Serve:** 4

- ¾ pound chicken tenders

- Prep + Cook Time2 whole eggs, beaten

- ½ cup seasoned breadcrumbs

- ½ cup all-purpose flour

- 1 tbsp black pepper

- 2 tbsp olive oil

1.Preheat your air fryer to 330 F. Add breadcrumbs, eggs and flour in three separate bowls (individually. Mix breadcrumbs with oil and season with salt and pepper. Dredge the tenders into flour, eggs and the crumbs.

2.Add chicken tenders in the Air Fryer and cook for 10 minutes. Increase to 390 F, and cook for 5 more minutes.

Chicken Tenders with Pineapple Juice

Prep Time: 4h 15 minutes | **Serve:** 4

- 1 lb boneless and skinless chicken tenders

- 4 cloves garlic, chopped

- 4 scallions, chopped

- 2 tbsp sesame seeds, toasted

- 1 tbsp fresh ginger, grated

- ½ cup pineapple juice

- ½ cup soy sauce

- ⅓ cup sesame oil

- A pinch of black pepper

1.Skew each tender and trim any excess fat. Mix the other ingredients in one large bowl. Add the skewered chicken and place in the fridge for 4 to 24 hours. Preheat the Air Fryer to 375°F.

2.Using a paper towel, pat the chicken until it is completely dry. Fry for 10 minutes.

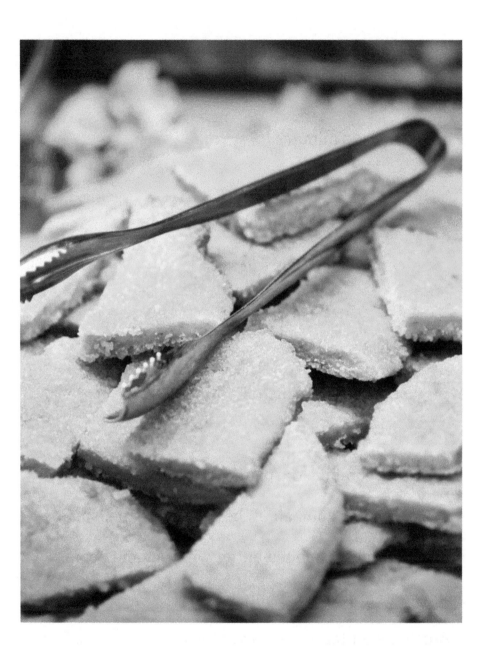

Crispy Panko Turkey Breasts

Prep Time: 25 minutes | **Serve:** 6

- 3 turkey breasts, boneless and skinless
- 2 cups panko1 tbsp salt
- ½ tsp cayenne pepper
- ½ tbsp black pepper
- 1 stick butter, melted

1.In a bowl, combine the panko, half of the black pepper, cayenne pepper, and half of the salt. In another small bowl, combine the melted butter with salt and pepper. Don't add salt if you use salted butter.

2.Brush the butter mixture over the turkey breasts. Coat the turkey with the panko mixture. Arrange them on a lined baking dish. Air fry for 15 minutes at 390 degrees F.

If the turkey breasts are thinner, cook only for 8 minutes.

Avocado-Mango Chicken Breasts

Prep Time: 3 hrs 20 minutes | **Serve:** 2

- 2 chicken breasts, cubed

- 1 large mango, cubed

- 1 medium avocado, sliced

- 1 red pepper, chopped

- 5 tbsp balsamic vinegar

- 15 tbsp olive oil

- 4 garlic cloves, minced

- 1 tbsp oregano

- 1 tbsp parsley, chopped

- A pinch of mustard powder

- Salt and black pepper to taste

1.In a bowl, mix whole mango, garlic, oil, and balsamic vinegar. Add the mixture to a blender and blend well. Pour the liquid over chicken cubes and soak for 3 hours. Take a pastry brush and rub the mixture over breasts as well.

2.Preheat your Air Fryer to 360 F. Place the chicken cubes in the cooking basket, and cook for 12 minutes. Add avocado, mango and pepper and toss well. Drizzle balsamic vinegar and garnish with chopped parsley.

Turkey Nuggets with Parsley & Thyme

Prep Time: 20 minutes | **Serve:** 2

- 8 oz turkey breast, boneless and skinless
- 1 egg, beaten
- 1 cup breadcrumbs
- 1 tbsp dried thyme
- ½ tbsp dried parsley
- Salt and black pepper to taste

1.Preheat the air fryer to 350 F. Mince the turkey in a food processor; transfer to a bowl. Stir in the thyme and parsley, and season with salt and pepper.

2.Take a nugget-sized piece of the turkey mixture and shape it into a ball, or another form. Dip in the breadcrumbs, then egg, then in the breadcrumbs again. Place the nuggets onto a prepared baking dish, and cook for 10 minutes.

Korean-Style Honey Chicken Wings

Prep Time: 15 minutes | **Serve:** 5

- 1 pound chicken wings

- 8 oz flour

- 8 oz breadcrumbs

- 3 beaten eggs

- 4 tbsp Canola oil

- Salt and black pepper to taste

- 2 tbsp sesame seeds

- 2 tbsp Korean red pepper paste

- 1 tbsp apple cider vinegar

- 2 tbsp honey

- 1 tbsp soy sauce

- Sesame seeds, to serve

1.Separate the chicken wings into winglets and drumettes. In a bowl, mix salt, oil and pepper. Preheat your Air Fryer to a temperature of 350 F. Coat the chicken with beaten eggs followed by breadcrumbs and flour.

2.Place the chicken in your Air Fryer's cooking basket. Spray with a bit of oil and cook for 15 minutes.

3.Mix red pepper paste, apple cider vinegar, soy sauce, honey and ¼ cup of water in a saucepan and bring to a boil over medium heat. Transfer the chicken to sauce mixture and toss to coat. Garnish with sesame to enjoy!

Savory Chicken Drumsticks with Honey and Garlic

Prep Time: 20 minutes | **Serve:** 3

- 2 chicken drumsticks, skin removed
- 2 tbsp olive oil
- 2 tbsp honey
- ½ tbsp garlic, minced

Preheat your Air Fryer to 400 F. Add garlic, oil and honey to a sealable zip bag. Add chicken and toss to coat; set aside for 30 minutes. Add the coated chicken to the Air Fryer basket, and cook for 15 minutes.

Garlic-Buttery Chicken Wings

Prep Time: 20 minutes | **Serve:** 4

- 16 chicken wings

- ¼ cup butter

- ¼ cup honey ½ tbsp salt

- 4 garlic cloves, minced ¾ cup potato starch

1.Preheat the air fryer to 370 F. Rinse and pat dry the wings, and place them in a bowl. Add the starch to the bowl, and mix to coat the chicken. Place the chicken in a baking dish that has been previously coated with cooking oil.

2.Cook for 5 minutes in the air fryer. Whisk the rest of the ingredients together in a bowl. Pour the sauce over the wings and cook for another 10 minutes.

Pineapple & Ginger Chicken Kabobs

Prep Time: 20 minutes | **Serve:** 4

- ¾ oz boneless and skinless chicken tenders ½ cup soy sauce
- ½ cup pineapple juice ¼ cup sesame oil
- 4 cloves garlic, chopped
- 1 tbsp fresh ginger, grated
- 4 scallions, chopped
- 2 tbsp toasted sesame seeds
- 1 A pinch of black pepper

1.Skewer the chicken pieces into the skewers and trim any fat. In a large sized bowl, mix the remaining ingredients.

2.Dip the skewered chicken into the seasoning bowl. Preheat your Air Fryer to 390 F. Pat the chicken to dry using a towel and place in the Air Fryer cooking basket. Cook for 5-7 minutes.

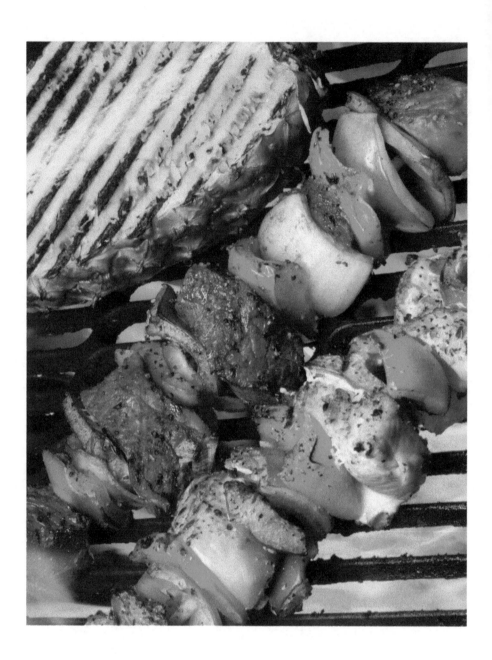

Worcestershire Chicken Breasts

Prep Time: 20 minutes | **Serve:** 6

- ¼ cup flour ½ tbsp flour

- 5 chicken breasts, sliced

- 1 tbsp Worcestershire sauce

- 3 tbsp olive oil

- ¼ cup onions, chopped

- 1 ½ cups brown sugar

- ¼ cup yellow mustard ¾ cup water

- ½ cup ketchup

1.Preheat your Fryer to 360 F. In a bowl, mix in flour, salt and pepper. Cover the chicken slices with flour mixture and drizzle oil over the chicken. In another bowl, mix brown sugar, water, ketchup, chopped onion, mustard, Worcestershire sauce and salt. Transfer chicken to marinade mixture; set aside for 10 minutes. Place the chicken in your Air Fryer's cooking basket and cook for 15 minutes.

Sherry Grilled Chicken

Prep Time: 25 minutes | **Serve:** 2

- 4 chicken breasts, cubed

- 2 garlic clove, minced

- ½ cup ketchup

- ½ tbsp ginger, minced

- ½ cup soy sauce

- 2 tbsp sherry

- ½ cup pineapple juice

- 2 tbsp apple cider vinegar

- ½ cup brown sugar

1.Preheat your Air Fryer to 360 F. In a bowl, mix in ketchup, pineapple Juice, sugar, cider vinegar, ginger.

Heat the sauce in a frying pan over low heat. Cover chicken with the soy sauce and sherry; pour the hot sauce on top. Set aside for 15 minutes to marinate. Place the chicken in the Air Fryer cooking basket and cook for 15 minutes.

Mustard Chicken with Thyme

Prep Time: 20 minutes | **Serve:** 4

- 4 garlic cloves, minced

- 8 chicken slices

- 1 tbsp thyme leaves

- ½ cup dry wine Salt as needed

- ½ cup Dijon mustard

- 2 cups breadcrumbs

- 2 tbsp melted butter

- 1 tbsp lemon zest

- 2 tbsp olive oil

1.Preheat your Air Fryer to 350 F. In a bowl, mix garlic,

salt, cloves, breadcrumbs, pepper, oil, butter and lemon

zest. In another bowl, mix mustard and wine. Place

chicken slices in the wine mixture and then in the crumb mixture. Place the prepared chicken in the Air Fryer cooking basket and cook for 15 minutes.

Shrimp Paste Chicken

Prep Time: 30 minutes | **Serve:** 2

- 8 chicken wings, washed and cut into small portions
- ½ tbsp sugar
- 2 tbsp corn flour
- ½ tbsp wine
- 1 tbsp shrimp paste
- 1 tbsp ginger
- ½ tbsp olive oil Directions

1.Preheat your Air Fryer to 360 F. In a bowl, mix oil, ginger, wine and sugar. Cover the chicken wings with the prepared marinade and top with flour. Add the floured chicken to shrimp paste and coat it.

2.Place the prepared chicken in your Air Fryer's cooking basket and cook for 20 minutes, until crispy on the outside.

Beef and Zucchinis Bowls

Prep Time: 10 min | **Cook Time:** 8 hours | **Serve:** 4

- 1 pound beef loin, cut into strips
- 1 tablespoon olive oil
- ¼ cup beef stock
- ½ teaspoon sweet paprika
- ½ teaspoon chili powder
- 2 small zucchinis, cubed
- 1 tablespoon balsamic vinegar
- 1 tablespoon chives, chopped

1.In your slow cooker, mix the beef with the oil, stock, and the other ingredients, toss, put the lid on and cook on Low for 8 hours.

2.Divide the mix between plates and serve.

Nutrition: 250 calories,31.1g protein, 2.4g

carbohydrates, 13.2g fat, 0.9g fiber, 81mg cholesterol,

121mg sodium, 566mg potassium.

Onion Beef with Olives

Prep Time: 10 min | **Cook Time:** 8 hours | **Serve:** 4

- 1 pound beef tenderloin, sliced

- ½ cup tomato passata

- 1 red onion, sliced

- 1 cup kalamata olives, pitted and halved

- Juice of ½ lime

- ¼ cup beef stock

- 1 tablespoon chives, hopped

1.In your slow cooker, mix the beef slices with the passata, onion, olives, and the other ingredients, toss, put the lid on and cook on Low for 8 hours.

2.Divide the mix between plates and serve.

Nutrition: 288 calories,33.8g protein, 5.5g carbohydrates, 14g fat, 1.7g fiber, 104mg cholesterol, 410mg sodium, 458mg potassium.

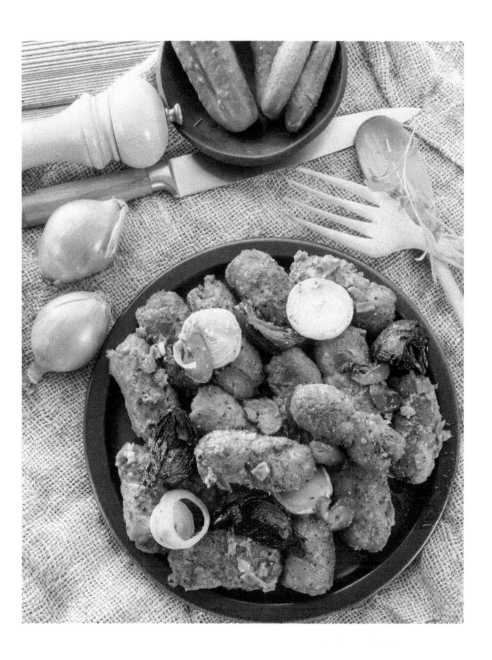

Beef Mix

Prep Time: 10 min | **Cook Time:** 8 hours | **Serve:** 4

- 1 pound beef loin, boneless and roughly cubed

- 3 tablespoons honey

- ½ tablespoons oregano, dried

- 1 tablespoon garlic, minced

- 1 tablespoon olive oil

- ½ cup beef stock

- ½ teaspoon sweet paprika

1.In your slow cooker, mix the beef loin with the honey, and the other ingredients, toss, put the lid on and cook on Low for 8 hours.

2.Divide everything between plates and serve.

Nutrition: 292 calories,31g protein, 14.2g

carbohydrates, 13.1g fat, 0.4g fiber, 81mg cholesterol,

161mg sodium, 434mg potassium.

Beef with Yogurt Sauce

Prep Time: 10 min | **Cook Time:** 8 hours | **Serve:** 4

- 1 pound beef loin, cubed

- 1 teaspoon garam masala

- ½ teaspoon turmeric powder

- 1 cup beef stock

- 1 teaspoon garlic, minced

- ½ cup Greek-style yogurt

- 1 tablespoon chives, chopped

1.In your slow cooker, mix the beef with the turmeric, garam masala, and the other ingredients, toss, put the lid on and cook on Low for 8 hours.

2.Divide everything into bowls and serve.

Nutrition: 228 calories,33.8g protein, 1.5g carbohydrates, 9.6g fat, 0.1g fiber, 82mg cholesterol, 269mg sodium, 469mg potassium.

Beans Mix with Meat

Prep Time: 10 min | **Cook Time:** 8 hours | **Serve:** 4

- 1 red bell pepper, chopped

- 1 pound beef loin, cubed

- 1 tablespoon olive oil

- 1 cup canned black beans, drained and rinsed ½ cup tomato sauce

- 1 yellow onion, chopped

- 1 teaspoon Italian seasoning

- 1 tablespoon oregano, chopped

1.In your slow cooker, mix the beef with the bell pepper, oil, and the other ingredients, toss, put the lid on and cook on Low for 8 hours.

2.Divide the mix between plates and serve.

Nutrition: 437 calories,41.9g protein, 37.6g

carbohydrates, 14.3g fat, 9.3g fiber, 81mg cholesterol,

228mg sodium, 1322mg potassium.

Beef and Spinach Bowls

Prep Time: 10 min | **Cook Time:** 7 hours | **Serve:** 4

- 1 red onion, sliced

- 1-pound beef loin, cubed

- 1 cup tomato passata

- 1 cup baby spinach

- 1 teaspoon olive oil

- ½ cup beef stock

- 1 tablespoon basil, chopped

1.In your slow cooker, mix the beef with the onion, passata, and the other ingredients except for the spinach, toss, put the lid on and cook on Low for 6 hours and 30 minutes.

2.Add the spinach, toss, put the lid on, cook on Low for 30 minutes more, divide into bowls, and serve.

Nutrition: 246 calories,31.7g protein, 4.5g

carbohydrates, 11.1g fat, 0.8g fiber, 81mg cholesterol,

94mg sodium, 470mg potassium.

Chilies Meat Mix

Prep Time: 10 min | **Cook Time:** 7 hours | **Serve:** 4

- 1 pound beef loin, cubed

- 1 tablespoon olive oil

- ½ green bell pepper, chopped

- 1 red onion, sliced

- ½ red bell pepper, chopped

- 1 garlic clove, minced

- 2 ounces canned green chilies, chopped ½ cup tomato passata

- 1 tablespoon chili powder

- 1 tablespoon cilantro, chopped

1.In your slow cooker, mix the beef with the oil, bell pepper, and the other ingredients, toss, put the lid on and cook on Low for 7 hours.

2.Divide into bowls and serve right away.

Nutrition: 263 calories,31.3g protein, 5.9g carbohydrates, 13.4g fat, 1.5g fiber, 81mg cholesterol, 83mg sodium, 494mg potassium.

Fragrant Tenderloin

Prep Time: 10 min | **Cook Time:** 8 hours | **Serve:** 2

- 2 beef tenderloin
- ½ cup tomato juice, fresh
- 1 tablespoon balsamic vinegar
- 1 tablespoon mustard
- 1 tablespoon chives, chopped

1.In your slow cooker, combine the meat with the tomato juice, and the other ingredients, toss, put the lid on, and cook on Low for 8 hours.

2.Divide between plates and serve with a side salad.

Nutrition: 214 calories,26.5g protein, 4.7g carbohydrates, 9.4g fat, 1.1g fiber, 78mg cholesterol, 214mg sodium, 491mg potassium.

Meat and Corn Mix

Prep Time: 10 min | **Cook Time:** 8 hours | **Serve:** 2

- 2 teaspoons olive oil

- 3 scallions, chopped

- 1 pound beef loin, cubed

- 1 cup of corn kernels

- ½ cup Greek-style yogurt

- ½ cup beef stock

- 2 garlic cloves, minced

- 1 tablespoon pomegranate sauce

- 1 tablespoon parsley, chopped

1.In your slow cooker, combine the beef with the corn, oil, scallions, and the other ingredients except for the yogurt, toss, put the lid on and cook on Low for 7 hours.

2.Add the yogurt, toss, cook on Low for 1 more hour,

divide into bowls and serve.

Nutrition: 284 calories,32.8g protein, 10.2g

carbohydrates, 13.3g fat, 1.5g fiber, 81mg cholesterol,

174mg sodium, 548mg potassium.

Lime Beef Mix

Prep Time: 10 min | **Cook Time:** 8 hours | **Serve:** 4

- 1 pound beef loin, cubed

- 1 tablespoon olive oil

- 3 garlic cloves, minced

- ½ yellow onion, chopped

- ½ cup beef stock

- 1 tablespoon apple cider vinegar

- 1 tablespoon lime zest, grated

1.In your slow cooker, mix the beef with the oil, garlic, and the other ingredients, toss, put the lid on, and cook on Low for 8 hours.

2.Divide everything between plates and serve.

Nutrition: 249 calories,31g protein, 2.3g carbohydrates, 13.1g fat, 0.5g fiber, 81mg cholesterol, 161mg sodium, 436mg potassium.

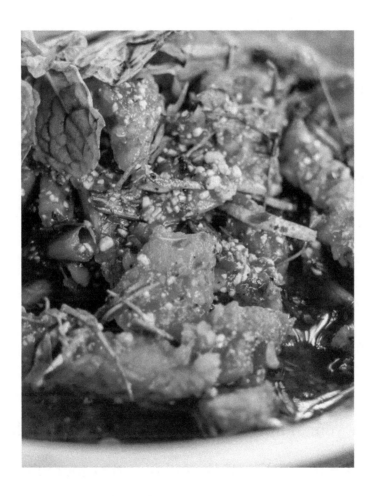

Coriander Beef Chops

Prep Time: 10 min | **Cook Time:** 6 hours | **Serve:** 4

- ½ pound beef chops
- ¼ tablespoons olive oil
- 2 garlic clove, minced
- ¼ teaspoon chili powder
- ½ cup beef stock
- ½ teaspoon coriander, ground
- ¼ teaspoon mustard powder
- 1 tablespoon tarragon, chopped

1.Grease your slow cooker with the oil and mix the beef chops with the garlic, stock, and the other ingredients inside.

2.Toss, put the lid on, cook on Low for 6 hours, divide between plates and serve with a side salad.

Nutrition: 204 calories,11.5g protein, 1.6g carbohydrates, 16.3g fat, 0.1g fiber, 44mg cholesterol, 456mg sodium, 41mg potassium.

Spicy Lime Beef Chops

Prep Time: 10 min | **Cook Time:** 5 hours | **Serve:** 4

- 2 teaspoons avocado oil

- 1 pound beef chops, bone-in

- 2 tablespoons mayonnaise, low-fat

- ½ tablespoon honey

- ¼ cup beef stock

- ½ tablespoon lime juice

1.In your slow cooker, mix the beef chops with the oil, honey, and the other ingredients, toss well, put the lid on, and cook on High for 5 hours.

2.Divide beef chops between plates and serve.

Nutrition: 253 calories,34.7g protein, 4.6g carbohydrates, 9.9g fat, 0.1g fiber, 103mg cholesterol, 177mg sodium, 480mg potassium.

Lightning Source UK Ltd.
Milton Keynes UK
UKHW020848180521
383917UK00001B/97